TEENAGE PREGNANCY

The Essential Guide

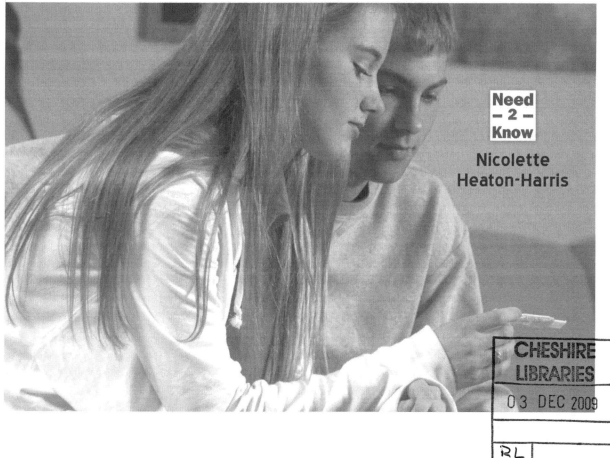

Need — 2 — Know

Nicolette
Heaton-Harris

First published in Great Britain in 2007 by
Need2Know
Remus House
Coltsfoot Drive
Peterborough
PE2 9JX
Telephone 01733 898105
Fax 01733 313524
www.need2knowbooks.co.uk

Need2Know is an imprint of Forward Press Ltd.
www.forwardpress.co.uk

Whilst every care has been taken to validate the contents of this
guide up to the time of going to press, the author advises that she
does not claim medical qualifications. The reader should seek
advice from a qualified medical practitioner before undertaking
any particular course of treatment, and similarly to take legal
advice as to the current state of any relevant laws in respect of
any matters contained herein.

Contents

Introduction

This book has been written to help navigate your way through many decisions and uncertainties that face you when you discover your daughter, a teenager, is pregnant.

This may not be what you wished for her, and understandably you may feel upset, angry or confused. But as her parent, your first priority should be for her, for getting all the information and help she'll need over the coming months, (years, if she decides to keep the baby.)

One in every 10 babies born in the United Kingdom today is born to a teenage girl. About 5% of under-18 conceptions are to young women aged under 15. They may think that they are ready to be parents and welcome the pregnancy, showing themselves to be happy and carefree, but they will still need your help, support and information, like any parent-to-be.

This book will clearly show you:

- How to know if your daughter is pregnant.

- How to prepare her for what is to come during pregnancy and birth.

- What she should expect.

- What a baby needs.

- How to help your daughter continue her education.

- The facts about abortion.

- What you need to know about adoption.

- Birth control.

- Further resources.

'1 in 10 babies is born to a teenager.'

'Sex, education, and teenage pregnancy.'

'She's little more than a baby herself.'

'Where can I turn for help and support?'

If your daughter has discovered she is pregnant, it does not have to be the end of the world. With support, knowledge and education the situation can have a happy outcome for all involved.

You can read this book straight through or just dip into the chapters you need as you require them, but keep it handy for guidance and, by all means, let your daughter read it too. It covers many topics, including pregnancy, birth, abortion and adoption. Each topic will be explained in detail so that you and your daughter (and the baby's father if he is involved) can make an *informed decision* about what they need and want to do. It is *their life.* They must choose and live with any decisions they make.

This book does not promote keeping the baby, abortion or adoption: its purpose is simply to give you information. Each option is discussed in a frank and factual way, as a choice open to your daughter.

- If she decides to keep the baby because it is the right thing for her, then so be it.

- If she decides to abort the baby because it is the right thing for her, then so be it.

- If she decides to have the baby adopted because it is the right thing for her, then so be it.

I hope this book will be invaluable, not only to parents of pregnant teenagers but also the expectant mother, the father-to-be, their families, teachers and professionals too.

With this book, you will be able to guide your loved ones through the minefield of choice and hard decisions on the understanding that you are doing everything you can for your daughter and her future.

Good luck and best wishes.

Chapter One
Is She Pregnant?

Do you suspect that your daughter is pregnant? Are there signs and suspicions that won't go away? Are you worried about what's going to happen to her future?

If the answer to these three questions is 'yes', you need to carefully work through these issues with your daughter, knowing that along the way there are going to be tears and strong emotions.

It can be a shock to even *suspect* that she may be pregnant. This is your daughter. You may feel she is little more than a child herself and be unsure of what to do or say.

So what is the answer?

Simply put, you have to learn as much as possible about the whole process. Arm yourself and your daughter with knowledge so that you can establish firm lines of communication for the coming months, knowing then that she will be able to turn to you with any fears and concerns and won't try to hide them away or do something alone that she may later regret.

You must remain as calm as you can, even if you feel like exploding with anger. It's not going to help anyone if you lose your temper, and it certainly won't encourage your daughter to talk to you. She's going to be scared enough, without you losing your rag. This is not to say that you don't have a right to be upset and angry. Of course you do. It's probably not what you wanted for your daughter, but you're going to have to contain these strong emotions until moments when you are not with her.

'Pregnancy tests are available from Brook Centres, family planning clinics, your daughter's GP and chemists.'

Early pregnancy symptoms

- Cessation of periods.

- Nausea and/or vomiting.

- Tender breasts.

- Frequent urination.

- Mood swings.

- Tiredness.

- Strange taste in the mouth.

How to find out for sure

First you need to know for certain. You have your suspicions but you now need proof. If your suspicions are correct, the earlier your daughter receives good medical care, the better – no matter what she decides to do.

She may already have approached you with her concerns, in which case you are lucky. Many young girls in the same situation ignore the signs, honestly thinking that if they ignore them then it might all go away, or it isn't really happening. If she has come to you, you should feel fortunate that you have such a good relationship.

Some girls may be afraid of their parent's reactions, worried that they might be letting them down in some way or that they may be furious.

The last thing you want is for your daughter to worry about this on her own, so open up and encourage her to communicate with you.

If she hasn't come to you, you might be tempted to ask her directly, especially if you're feeling angry, shocked or let down. A better way might be to open up a general conversation, somewhere private like her bedroom, and work it round to your worries and suspicions.

Just remember, no matter how you feel about it, she will be feeling just as scared and anxious as you. Take a few moments to breathe deeply and stay calm. Shouting and yelling angry remarks will not help and may make things worse.

You are the adult. Show her that you care (even if you're furious) and that you want to help. Ask her what symptoms she's had, whether she's seen a doctor and if she's taken a home pregnancy test.

Are home pregnancy tests reliable?

The answer is 'yes'. The tests are very accurate and there is very little risk of a 'false positive' result. It is always best to purchase a kit that contains two tests, so that if the first is negative, a second test can be performed a week later to confirm the correct result.

Home kits work by detecting human chorionic gonadotrophin (HCG) which is produced in the body when a pregnancy implants in the lining of the womb. HCG can be detected in a blood test as early as six days after conception, but for a home pregnancy testing kit, which relies on your daughter producing a urine sample, you have to wait two to three weeks after conception or on the first day of your missed period. The more sensitive the pregnancy test is, the earlier it will show a positive result.

OK. It's definite. What do we do now?

If your concerns are confirmed then you need to take your daughter to a GP who will give her a general health check and test for pregnancy, if she hasn't used a home test herself. Remember that some early symptoms of pregnancy can be due to other medical conditions.

It may take a day or two for the results to come back, depending upon the doctor's method of testing, but you can use this time effectively to talk with your daughter. See how she feels, what her immediate thoughts are and if there is anything she needs. She may even tell you who the baby's father is and what his role in this might be.

Chapter Two
Decisions

Once the pregnancy has been confirmed, you're going to have to help your daughter make some tough decisions, and there are no easy options.

She has three choices facing her and must choose one of them:

- Have an abortion.

- Have the baby adopted.

- Keep the baby.

It may seem harsh set out so clearly and bluntly, but this is the reality of the situation. Each option must be thought through properly and thoroughly for the sake of your daughter's future.

It may help to break each of the three choices into sets of questions that she can ask herself and discuss with you. I have listed the main ones below, but as you discuss them with her you may think of others, and this is fine too.

If she decides:

To have an abortion

- Does she understand what happens?

- Can her family and friends support her afterwards?

- Does she realise that an abortion can be traumatic?

- Does she feel that this is the *right choice for her?*

To have the baby adopted

- Does she know the different types of adoption?

- What type would she prefer?

- Does she want the child to know who she is?

- Does she want to maintain contact with the adoptive family?

- Can she go through birth and give the baby away?

- Does she feel like this is the *right choice for her?*

To keep the baby

- Will she be able to look after the baby herself?

- Can she be responsible for this new life for the next 20 years?

- Will she want to continue her education with a baby to care for?

- Will the baby's father, or his family, be involved?

- Will her family and friends support her?

- Can she afford a baby?

- Where will she live?

- Does she feel this is the *right choice for her?*

You may notice that the final question in each choice is the same.

Is this the right choice for her?

This is very important. The end decision must be your daughter's. You can listen and give advice as you see things but in the end you cannot tell her what she must do, no matter how much you may want to persuade her. You may worry about her future and feel that she will ruin her life by having a child but you shouldn't force her into adoption or abortion. In the same way, you shouldn't try to persuade her into keeping the baby just because you would like a grandchild.

It's her choice. The decision must rest with her alone. This seems a big thing for someone who is so young, but she is the one who will have to live with this decision for the rest of her life. If you have been responsible for persuading her, you will also be partly to blame if things don't go well.

If you can contain any strong feelings you may have and spend time helping her to talk decisions through, you will at least know that you did the right thing by giving her the support she needed and a shoulder to cry on.

And *she* will know it too. You don't want her to turn on you in future years saying everything is *your fault* because *you told her what to do.*

Who do we tell?

Should you tell anyone in the early stages?

This is very much down to personal choice, but there are many people you may consider telling. If your daughter is experiencing some of the symptoms of early pregnancy, it may be difficult to avoid suspicion and questions.

Think about telling:

- Your daughter's school.

- The baby's father.

- The rest of the family.

You may not think it is necessary to tell the school. This is up to you and your daughter but, if she is suffering with sickness or tiredness, they can make allowances for this if they know.

When I was at school, a 13-year-old girl in my class got pregnant. The school allowed her to sit out of PE lessons and any science/chemistry classes which included using chemicals. She was also allowed to eat/drink in class whenever she needed, and they made allowances for her visits to the doctor and antenatal appointments. These might seem of low significance but they were important to the girl and her family, and it might be worth thinking about them at this stage. Would it help your daughter if the school knew?

The baby's father

Of course, on discovering the pregnancy, you're going to wonder who the father of the baby is. If your daughter has a boyfriend you know about then he may be the obvious candidate, but if there isn't a boyfriend you will need to handle this situation carefully.

You will want to establish that she had intercourse willingly and wasn't forced in any way.

Although you may have many questions, your daughter might not want to tell you who he is. If this is the case, then leave it for now, you don't need to get into any upsetting arguments. Your daughter will probably tell you when she is ready. Be sure to tell her how much you care, and that you're only asking because you love her, not because you want to confront him and read the riot act.

Explain that:

- If she decides to keep the baby, doctors and midwives will want to know the father's medical history as well as her own.

- He has a right (and responsibility) to know about the baby and be given the chance to be involved with the child he has helped create.

- If your daughter decides to have the baby adopted, the adoptive family will want to know the medical history of both birth parents.

Telling the father-to-be and his family may be a tempestuous event. Try and remain calm and, as ever, keep those lines of communication open. Perhaps you could arrange a time to visit him with your daughter and suggest that everyone remain seated while you talk about what has happened. There may be some volatile reactions. There may be stunned silence or disbelief. You may even be accused of lying. Who knows how they will react? Just keep reiterating that you are ready to answer their questions when they want to talk calmly, because tension and upset will not help anyone.

Questions

There are many questions in people's minds at this stage and you would be advised to spend time with your daughter, prompting her to think about some topics she might not have thought of herself. Questions such as:

- If she keeps the baby, what will she have to give up in her life and is that okay?

- What had she wanted for her future before the pregnancy?

- Will having a baby prevent those aims?

- Does her pregnancy interfere with her religious beliefs?

- Has she thought about life as a single parent?

Checklist

- Find out for sure if she's pregnant.

- Start thinking and talking about the options.

- See a doctor.

- Ask about the father.

- Tell those who need to know.

- Keep lines of communication open.

Chapter Three

Abortion?

Your daughter may decide that the best thing is to have an abortion. You may agree with her, or you may be upset at her choice, but you must keep your lines of communication open and not force her into something she may resent you for at a later date.

Choosing an abortion, like her other options, is an enormous decision. You'll want to make sure that she understands her choice and all the implications of it.

What happens?

There are different ways an abortion can be carried out, depending upon how far pregnant your daughter is.

A medical history will be taken, and legal requirements ensure that the abortion process is fully explained.

An ultrasound scan will be performed to check how many weeks pregnant she is, and to ensure the baby is growing within the womb and not ectopic (where the pregnancy grows outside of the uterus, such as in a fallopian tube).

Next, the clinic will perform a blood test for routine checks including her blood group and Rhesus factor.

A urine test may also be performed.

Legalities

At the time of writing, termination of pregnancy before 24 weeks of gestation is legal in the UK. However, many hospitals and clinics will not consider termination beyond 18 to 20 weeks, so it is therefore advisable to discuss this with her GP sooner rather than later. Termination after 24 weeks may be legal in certain circumstances, according to the *Amendments to the Abortion Act 1967* and *1991* (Britain only).

If your daughter chooses to have an abortion, she should have support from those around her and counselling before and after the procedure.

Two doctors must agree to terminate the pregnancy, basing their decision on the following:

- Continuing the pregnancy would be riskier than terminating it, causing harm to the physical or mental health of the mother-to-be.

- Termination is required to prevent serious harm and injury to the mental/physical health of the mother-to-be.

- Continuing the pregnancy would put the mother's life at risk.

- There is risk that if the child was born it would suffer serious physical or mental handicap.

There are two further clauses which have to be adhered to:

- That the pregnancy is not beyond the 24th week and that continuing the pregnancy would involve risk for the mother.

- That the pregnancy has not exceeded the 24th week and that continuing the pregnancy would involve substantial mental/physical harm to existing children of the mother or her family.

Induced abortion

- In the first three months, abortion may be carried out using a vacuum technique. This is done under general anaesthetic, local anaesthetic or heavy sedation.

- If the pregnancy is less than 63 days from your daughter's last period, medical staff may use a prostaglandin pessary in the vagina, along with a tablet called mifepristone by mouth.

- From the fourth to the sixth month of pregnancy more detailed methods are employed. Labour contractions are induced and your daughter will experience pains which may last some time.

If your daughter is found to be Rhesus negative, she will be given anti-D immunoglobulin after the pregnancy has come away. This prevents her from developing troublesome antibodies in future pregnancies.

Infection is a possibility after any abortion, no matter what stage of the pregnancy, so antibiotics may be given following any of these procedures.

Your daughter should be given a single room so that she can have privacy at all times during the procedure. The medical staff should explain what is happening at each stage.

Parental consent?

You may think that your daughter requires your consent to have an abortion, but she does not. If she has told her school before you, the teachers and social services can arrange for her to see a doctor and they are not obliged to tell you about it. This can seem quite unfair but, at the time of writing, this is the law as it stands.

Counselling

Grief and upset following a termination is common. Even if your daughter knows that she had an abortion for all the right reasons, she can still get incredibly upset at what she has done and been through.

Aftercare

Aftercare advice should be given and *followed*. If your daughter is tearful, either from grief or overwhelming relief, it may fall to you to remind her about what she should do to prevent an infection afterwards.

'A private abortion costs from around £450. Prices increase dramatically the more advanced the pregnancy is. See Brook or BPAS in the help list.'

Some centres, like Marie Stopes clinics, provide counsellors if your daughter feels she needs to talk to someone outside of her immediate family. They have a 24 hour aftercare advice line: 0845 1221441.

Your emotions

Sometimes you, members of the family, can feel a sense of grief too, and it's easy to overlook this as all the attention has been focused on your daughter. This can come from feelings of loss of a grandchild, but can also be from feeling unable to protect your daughter from physical and mental pain, grief and loss.

Try to talk together about what has happened, but be sensitive to times when your daughter may not want to speak. If necessary, speak to a counsellor, your doctor, or a trusted friend if you need to share these strong emotions with someone else.

'It is possible to become pregnant again very soon after having an abortion. It is never too early to start thinking about contraception – even if your daughter thinks she won't be having sex ever again!'

Chapter Four
Adoption?

What is adoption?

Adoption is the legal process of giving up a baby to be parented by another person or persons.

If your daughter feels that this is the best choice for her, then she will have to navigate her way through a lot of legal requirements and paperwork.

There will be decisions about what kind of adoption she wants:

- Does she want to give up the baby and have no contact whatsoever?
- Would she like the authorities to register the fact that she would be happy to be contacted in the future?

What happens?

If adoption is chosen, a social worker will talk over the decision to adopt with your daughter. They will want to make sure that she knows what she is doing, what it means, and that she fully understands the future implications of her choice.

Consent

Your daughter will not be able to sign any papers regarding adoption until the baby is over six weeks of age. She may choose to care for her baby during this time (which can increase the possibility of her changing her mind as she becomes attached to the baby) or she can have the baby placed into foster care.

An agency or the social services will choose the best people to adopt the baby. (Families that wish to adopt babies and children go through many checks to help ensure they will make suitable parents.)

Future contact?

Your daughter will have the right to contact the adoptive parents at the time or in the future. Sometimes limited contact can be agreed upon, but this has to be the choice of everyone involved. (Everyone includes the new adoptive parents, your daughter, you and social services.)

When the baby reaches 18, he/she will be entitled by law to obtain their original birth certificates and adoption papers. This is another reason to consider whether your daughter places the name of the baby's father on the certificate. Will he be happy to be contacted at some point in the future?

The idea of future contact is an important one. Your daughter may not worry too much about it now, but how will she feel in 18 years time? She may be married and have other children when the adopted child turns up to find her.

- How will she deal with this?

- Has she thought about what to say?

- Does she want to write a letter she can leave with the adoption papers for her child to read when they come of age?

Counselling

Giving a baby up for adoption is usually an incredibly difficult and emotional experience and certainly could not be described as easy.

Having carried the baby for nine months and experienced the trials of labour and birth, many women find they are so strongly attached to their babies that adoption is not for them.

In this situation, the social workers will be at hand to talk to your daughter and discuss her options. She may also be offered a counsellor.

As her parent you should try to spend whatever time with her that she needs, in a supportive and loving capacity.

Decision to go ahead with adoption

If your daughter still wishes to place the baby up for adoption, you and social services will want to make sure that she has asked herself a few searching questions.

- Can she face giving the baby away having gone through pregnancy, labour and birth?

- Can she cope with not knowing what is happening to her baby?

- Will she be able to cope with other people's comments and possible gossip?

- How will she feel if the child appears on her doorstep, years into the future?

- Is the baby's father for or against the adoption?

Information

If your daughter feels she has many unresolved issues, or you want to ask questions about what is happening, there are organisations that can help you both.

Adoption Info Line (9am-9pm, except bank holidays)
204 Stockport Road, Altrincham, WA15 7UA
Tel: 0800 783 4086
www.adoption.org.uk

Talk Adoption (Confidential helpline)
12 Chapel Street, Manchester, M3 7NH
Tel: 0808 808 1234 (Tues-Fri, 3pm-9pm)
www.talkadoption.org.uk
helpline@talkadoption.org.uk

'Even if your daughter is sure adoption is the right choice for her, she's likely to experience a range of emotions including guilt, loss, grief and low self-esteem. Remember these feelings may surface straight away or not until months - even years later.'

Checklist

- Talk.

- Decide about future contact.

- Discuss options with social services.

- Ensure you know what is happening at every stage.

- Make sure your daughter is certain this is what she wants.

Chapter Five

Healthy Pregnancy

Teenage mothers

The government's Social Exclusion Report, 1999, states: 'experiencing a pregnancy during teenage years could have an extremely detrimental effect on the young parents and their subsequent baby'.

What are the disadvantages?

- It was suggested that teenagers are disadvantaged by a lack of complete education as most teenage mothers fail to return to education after the birth. This affects their chances of gaining employment in the future and any subsequent career choices.

- There is a greater risk to their health. Teenage mothers are more likely to suffer complications such as anaemia, pre-eclampsia and complications of labour.

- There is a greater risk to the baby. It was deemed more likely to be of low birth weight (25% higher chance than other mothers), and there is a noted higher infant mortality rate in teenage mothers (almost 60% higher than other mothers).

- A teenage mother is also three times more likely to suffer post-natal depression.

Having said this, it does not mean that your daughter or her baby will be affected by these statistics. She may have a very healthy pregnancy with no complications before, during or after the birth. She may continue her education and go on in future years to gain sound employment with good future

'Most areas have a specialist teenage pregnancy midwife. There may even be antenatal and parentcraft classes especially for teenage parents. Your daughter can ask her GP/midwife or contact Connexions for details.'

prospects. Just because she is a teenage mother does not mean she is some statistic, doomed to fail in life. That is the stereotype. But we can change that with support and more focus on education.

With these statistics in mind, many maternity units have established teenage antenatal clinics, and these run parentcraft classes too.

Sure Start, an initiative introduced by the government in 1999, helps with these and other problems. It is worth (no matter what your daughter's decision) finding out where your nearest Sure Start Plus provider is.

Staying healthy

When most women plan to have a family they try to ensure their health and lifestyle is as good as it possibly can be before conception. This is the best way.

In the case of teenagers, where pregnancy is often unplanned, young girls may not have prepared their bodies for the physical task that lies ahead. In this situation, the only thing a young mother-to-be can do is ensure she eats a healthy diet and lives a healthy lifestyle as soon as she discovers the pregnancy.

Dieting

Reducing calorie intake while carrying a baby is not a wise thing to do; pregnancy is not the time to try to lose weight. However, if your daughter feels that in the early months she can only consume certain foods because of feelings of nausea or sickness, she should not worry too much about this.

Nausea and vomiting

In over half of all pregnancies there are signs of nausea and vomiting in the mother-to-be. No-one knows exactly what causes it, but there are many different suggestions on how to deal with it. Your daughter could try:

- Eating a dry biscuit before getting out of bed.

- Eating frequently during the day.

- Avoiding spicy foods.

- Eating small amounts frequently.

- Eating ginger or ginger biscuits.

- Sucking on boiled sweets, such as barley sugar.

Healthy eating

If your daughter was underweight before getting pregnant, she has a higher chance of anaemia and carrying a low birth-weight baby.

If she was overweight, then she has a higher risk of being affected by gestational diabetes and blood pressure problems.

In the UK today, people eat too much fat in their diet. This is a well-known fact. Newspapers and magazines abound with dieting advice.

But what about advice on a normal, healthy diet?

Information is available from the Food Standards Agency who advise that we eat more starchy foods such as cereals and bread, as well as plenty of fruit and vegetables, at least five portions per day.

Eating healthily on a low budget can be difficult. Take advantage of highly nutritious yet cheap foods, such as jacket potatoes and salad or baked beans. There are also various types of pasta which can be mixed with vegetables or a tin of tuna fish.

She does not need to 'eat for two'. In fact, in the final three months of pregnancy, a pregnant woman only needs to eat an extra 250-500 calories a day.

'Healthy eating doesn't have to be complicated. Have at least five portions of fruit or vegetables each day. Choose wholegrain bread, rice, pasta, etc. Limit high fat and sugar foods such as cakes and biscuits. Choose lean cuts of meat. Try and eat at least two servings of fish per week.'

Vitamin A

There are many different vitamins and minerals that are essential to health, and when your daughter sees her doctor or midwife she will be advised on a healthy diet.

It is of paramount importance that she does not consume too much Vitamin A. This does not mean she is not allowed it at all as Vitamin A helps to build up resistance to infection and it strengthens tooth enamel, but if she consumes a large amount it may increase her chances of having a baby with a birth defect. Vitamin A can be found in:

'Avoid eating shark and swordfish, and limit tuna to two steaks (or four cans) per week. This is because of concerns about mercury levels.'

- Whole milk.

- Egg yolk.

- Oily fish.

- Liver.

- Green and yellow vegetables.

- Carrots.

Other vitamins and minerals

Vitamin B1
Found in whole grains, nuts, liver, brewer's yeast and wheat germ. Helps with digestion and keeping the stomach lining and intestines healthy.

Vitamin B2
Found in brewer's yeast, wheat germ, whole grains, green vegetables, liver, eggs and milk. Helps keep eyes and skin healthy.

Vitamin B6
Found in whole grains, liver, mushrooms, potatoes and bananas. Helps the body's immune system. A lack of it can contribute towards anaemia.

- **Vitamin B12**

  Found in whole grains, milk and fish. Helps our red blood cells to develop and is important for the baby's nervous system.

- **Vitamin C**

  Found in citrus fruits such as oranges, lemons and limes, and some vegetables. (It can be destroyed by cooking so it is best to eat these foods in their raw state. As we cannot store vitamin C it needs to be replaced each day.) Helps our immune system to fight infection. It also aids with the healthy growth of the baby's placenta.

- **Vitamin D**

  Absorbed from sunshine, found in oil and eggs. Helps to build and strengthen our bones.

- **Vitamin E**

  Found in most foods.

- **Vitamin K**

  Found in green leafy vegetables. Important to assist normal clotting mechanisms of blood. Most babies will be automatically injected with vitamin K after birth, with the mother's permission.

- **Calcium**

  Found in milk, cheese and fish. Helps to build and strengthen bones.

- **Iron**

  Found in beans, apricots, egg yolks and red meats. Essential during pregnancy in maintaining the quality of oxygen carrying blood cells.

- **Niacin**

  Found in eggs, milk, oily fish, brewer's yeast and green vegetables. Helps build our brain cells. Can also help if bleeding gums are a problem.

- **Zinc**

  Found in eggs, nuts, wheat and shellfish.

'If your daughter is vegetarian or vegan she may need to take extra care that she is getting all of her vitamins. Her doctor or midwife can advise.'

- **Folic acid**

  Rich sources of folate are found in many foods such as cabbages, fruit, beans, yeast extract and folate-rich breakfast cereals. This B-complex vitamin will probably be prescribed on confirmation of your daughter's pregnancy. Its function in helping development of the neural tube of the baby is well known. Folic acid tablets are usually only prescribed for the first three months of pregnancy.

Foods to avoid

- Soft and blue-veined cheeses.

- Unpasteurised milk or cheese.

- Shellfish.

- Raw egg foods, e.g. mayonnaise.

- Pâté.

- Undercooked meat.

- Liver (not more than one portion per week because of its high vitamin A content).

Food precautions

Any food you buy for your daughter should be from a reputable source, especially if it has already been prepared. Cook all foods thoroughly, especially if you've had to reheat them.

Other food safety rules apply. Wash all fruit and vegetables thoroughly and check that the temperature of your fridge is below 4°C. If your daughter is invited to a barbecue, ensure that anything she eats is cooked thoroughly and that all salads have been washed.

Exercise

There is no reason why your daughter should cease to exercise when she discovers she is pregnant. Moderate exercise has been shown to be very beneficial in an uncomplicated pregnancy and can even help when it's time for delivery. If she has any worries then it would be best to ask her doctor or midwife's advice.

If she becomes extremely fatigued or exhausted during any exercise activity, she should stop at once and ensure that she keeps up her fluid and energy intake.

Smoking

By the time they are 16, many teenagers smoke or have tried smoking. If your daughter is a smoker and wants to keep the baby or give it up for adoption, she must be encouraged and supported to cease smoking for her own health and that of the baby.

The baby growing in the womb depends on your daughter for everything. All its nutrients and oxygen come via the placenta and umbilical cord, which are damaged by smoking.

The baby is also exposed to toxins and carbon monoxide from tobacco smoke.

In some cases, the baby struggles to get enough oxygen. This can have serious or disastrous results as there is an increased risk of the baby's placenta becoming so damaged that it comes away from the womb before the baby is born (placental abruption). This may cause the baby to be born prematurely, starved of oxygen or even to die in the womb.

'Some research suggests caffeine may be harmful in pregnancy. Switch to caffeine-free alternatives where possible.'

Smoking facts

Babies born to mothers who smoke:

- Are frequently smaller in birth weight (see *the big myth* overleaf). During their first year, the more the mother smokes, the less the baby weighs.

- Have an increased risk of developing asthma.

- Are twice as likely to die of Sudden Infant Death Syndrome (SIDS).

- Are slower at school in learning to read.

- Are more likely to be born prematurely.

- Have organs that are smaller on average than babies born to non-smokers.

- Have poorer lung function.

- Are ill more frequently. Babies born to women who smoked 15 cigarettes or more a day during pregnancy are taken into hospital twice as often during the first eight months of life.

- Get painful diseases such as inflammation of the middle ear and asthmatic bronchitis more frequently in early childhood.

- Are more likely to become smokers themselves in later years.

> 'Try to smoke only outside and ask smoking visitors to do the same.'

> 'Never smoke in a child's bedroom.'

> 'Don't smoke while you are washing, dressing or playing with a child.'

> 'Never smoke in the car if there are children in it.'

The big myth

Many young (and older) mothers-to-be believe that if they smoke in pregnancy the baby will be smaller and everything will be easier.

What a serious mistake this is when you consider all the potential complications above.

It's sad to realise that whereas legislation increasingly protects children from parental cruelty, there's nothing to protect them from this while they're still in the womb.

If your daughter smokes and feels that she will have difficulty in giving it up, she can be referred for appropriate help through the NHS Quit Smoking Helpline. An advisor will give her advice and details of local groups. She can then be helped to give up by herself or with support from other quitters.

Alcohol

Drinking while pregnant is not advised. There is some debate as to whether a single glass of wine occasionally might be safe, but if in doubt, don't do it. Remember, alcohol is a drug.

Babies born to mothers who drink heavily can suffer with Foetal Alcohol Syndrome and be quite severely damaged.

Sexual health

If your daughter is pregnant, her doctor will probably want her to attend a sexual health clinic to check for STIs (sexually transmitted infections), whether or not she and her partner used a condom.

If they used condoms, her risk will be reduced although there is obviously still some risk: if sperm got through so could infection.

If she never used any form of protection and had more than one partner, then her chances of infection are high. Most teenagers are notorious for thinking that nothing bad can happen to them, but it can. So if the doctor suggests this visit, it is advisable for your daughter's health and future fertility that she goes. Remember, some sexually transmitted infections don't always show signs of infection (such as chlamydia). See *Sexually Transmitted Infections –The Essential Guide* for further information.

Other medical conditions

You may be worrying if your daughter has another condition to deal with as well as a pregnancy. How might diabetes or epilepsy affect her and the baby?

Diabetes

Diabetes can worsen during pregnancy, but with regular monitoring and check-ups, your daughter should be well cared for. This is why it is so important that she attends all her check-ups and appointments.

'17,000 children under five are admitted to hospital each year with illnesses resulting from passive smoking.'

'85% of cigarette smoke is invisible.'

Epilepsy

One third of epileptic women will experience more seizures while pregnant. This is because anti-epilepsy medications are reduced to the lowest possible dose during pregnancy. You should both ask your midwife and doctor about any concerns you may have in these cases.

Chapter Six

Antenatal Care

Both you and your daughter need to know what happens in the next few months. I know you've probably had a child yourself, but things are likely to have changed since you were pregnant. It may even be that your daughter is not your biological child and that you have never experienced pregnancy.

I'll cover the basics and what you'll both need to know, but if you need to look into things in more detail, then do not hesitate to ask the doctor or midwife.

Visiting the doctor

Your daughter is certainly going to get asked lots of questions, most of which will be medical. You can both use this opportunity to ask any questions of your own too. If you forget anything, don't worry, there'll be plenty more appointments with medical staff over the next few months.

What will she be asked?

- Is she going ahead with the pregnancy?

- When was the first day of her last menstrual period (LMP)?

- Numerous questions about her health history.

- Is she taking folic acid?

- What sort of antenatal care and birth would she like?

- Is she suffering with any pregnancy symptoms?

'Doctors, nurses and other health workers are not allowed to give out information about patients unless they think they're in danger, even if a patient is under 16.'
'Workers are more likely to be worried about young people under 13 who are having sex.'
'You can ring a surgery or clinic beforehand if you are worried about what may or may not be kept private.'

First trimester (first 12 weeks)

The first three months of your daughter's pregnancy is likely to be a roller-coaster of emotions and physical changes. These are entirely normal.

Minor disorders

Below is a list of commonly experienced minor disorders of the first 12 weeks of pregnancy:

- Abdominal twinges (anything prolonged should be investigated).

- Backache (anything prolonged should be investigated).

- Bleeding gums.

- Breast tenderness.

- Constipation.

- Cravings.

- Fainting or feeling light-headed.

- Increased flatulence.

- Insomnia.

- Frequency of passing urine. (If this is painful, it could be due to infection. The doctor should be consulted.)

- Morning sickness.

- Nasal sensitivity.

- Difference in taste.

- Thrush.

- Tiredness.

- Increased vaginal discharge.

- Varicose veins.

- Visual disturbances.

The list sounds terrible, but reassure your daughter that she might not experience any of these, or she may just experience some. Her body is flooding with hormones and physical changes are occurring internally and externally.

But what is happening to the baby?

The baby

In the first trimester, the baby will grow from a cluster of almost invisible cells into a miniature human being, measuring about three inches long and weighing as much as a pound coin. Most of the baby's internal organs will have developed by the end of this trimester, and its muscles are working so it can move about, although your daughter will not be aware of movements at this stage.

Most miscarriages occur in this first stage of pregnancy and your daughter should know about this risk. Ask her to be aware of her own body. If she experiences abdominal or back pain she should let you or a doctor know immediately. She should also report shoulder tip pain as this can be a sign of ectopic pregnancy (when the pregnancy grows elsewhere, such as in a fallopian tube).

At the end of the 12 weeks, your daughter will be invited for a 'booking visit' with the midwife, and in a separate appointment she will probably have her first scan at the hospital.

The booking visit

At this visit your daughter will be introduced to one of the midwives who will care for her throughout her pregnancy. She will be asked about her health history and also about that of the baby's father and his family, if she knows it. She will be told about local parentcraft classes, and it is advisable that she books into these as soon as she can as places fill fast. The midwife may also advise her about a tour of the hospital's delivery suite. These tours can be very helpful for a nervous, new mum-to-be.

Other things that may be done are:

- Blood pressure.
- Bloods test.
- Urine test.
- Height and weight.

She is also likely to be asked about the following:

- Her menstrual history.
- Birth preferences and pain relief.
- Feeding preferences.
- Her religious belief.
- If there is a history of multiple birth in the family.
- Is she currently on any medication?
- Any other risk factors.

What is the blood test for?

These are for:

- Blood group and Rhesus factor (in case she were to need a blood transfusion or Anti-D Immunoglobulin to prevent Rhesus antibodies).
- Haemoglobin (iron) levels (to determine whether she needs to take iron or not).

Less obvious checks:

'Toxoplasmosis is a common infection, dangerous to pregnant women and their babies. It is mostly passed on through cat faeces. Pregnant women should avoid changing cat litter trays (and take care when gardening in case there are faeces in the soil).'

- Syphilis.

- Rubella.

- Sickle cell disease.

- Hepatitis 'B'.

- Toxoplasmosis.

Your daughter may be offered a test for HIV/AIDS. Antenatal staff are unlikely to provide more than the most basic of explanations as to what a positive test result could mean. It is a good idea to contact your local HIV social worker or specialist agency prior to taking the test if there is any chance the result could come back positive.

Why do the tests?

As well as checking your daughter's health, the midwife will be on the lookout for any signs that things are not going well.

These can include:

- Haemoglobin lower than 10 g/dl (anaemia).

- Underweight or overweight.

- High blood pressure.

- Womb not growing to the correct size for the number of weeks/months.

- Any bleeding.

- Signs of infection.

- Any illness.

- Social or psychological risk factors.

She may be given her notes at this appointment, but usually they are given at 20 weeks after the anomaly scan.

'If you live on a farm, don't let your daughter handle lambing ewes, their afterbirth, newborn lambs or the clothing of anyone involved in the lambing as toxoplasmosis is also quite common in sheep.'

Medical abbreviations

If your daughter reads her notes, she will see that medical staff use a lot of abbreviation. Some of the more frequent ones are explained below:

- NAD   Nothing abnormal detected.

- MSU   Midstream urine sample.

- BP   Blood pressure.

- FH   Foetal heart.

- FHH   Foetal heart heard.

- LMP   Last menstrual period.

- EDD   Estimated date of delivery.

- Hb   Haemoglobin (iron) levels.

- Fe   Iron (tablets).

- FMF   Foetal movements felt.

- FMNF Foetal movements not felt.

- Vx/Ceph Vertex or Cephalic (baby is head down).

- Br   Breech (baby is bottom down).

- Eng   Whether the baby's head has engaged in the pelvis.

- NE   Not engaged.

Miscarriage

Miscarriage can occur at any time during a pregnancy, but most usually occur during the first trimester.

15% of pregnancies end in miscarriage. There are many reasons for this including abnormalities in the baby, infection, illness in the mother and environmental factors.

If your daughter experiences a miscarriage, it is vital that she understands that there was probably nothing she could have done to prevent it.

Whether the pregnancy was planned or not, a miscarriage is likely to be a big shock and she may need time to grieve. Make sure she knows it wasn't her fault. Some women who miscarry believe that they could have prevented it, but this is rarely the case.

Personally, I have experienced two miscarriages, both at six weeks of gestation. In both cases I was taking folic acid, eating healthily, not exposing myself to any dangers and was happy and content. Following confirmation of the pregnancies, I had the odd strong twinge of pain that worried me, but assumed this to be normal.

On the first occasion, I felt extreme prolonged pain low in my abdomen, about a minute in length. Minutes later, I noticed I was bleeding. I took myself to bed to rest, yet I lost the baby.

The second time, there were no pains at all. I just went to the toilet and noticed I was bleeding.

Early miscarriages can rarely be prevented. If they are going to happen, there is virtually nothing anyone can do to stop it.

Ectopic pregnancy

Signs that a pregnancy is ectopic usually occur before eight weeks.

The main signs to look out for are:

- Low abdominal pain.

- Vaginal bleeding/spotting.

- Shoulder pain.

'Quite a few women experience light bleeding some time in the first 12 weeks of pregnancy. Bleeding doesn't necessarily mean a miscarriage, but the GP/midwife should always be contacted for advice. If bleeding is heavy or pain is severe, call an ambulance or take your daughter to A&E. You can call NHS Direct on 0845 4647.'

- Nausea/vomiting.

- Dizziness.

First scan and tests

This first scan is a very special moment and one that first-time mums usually remember forever. Your daughter will be asked to arrive with a full bladder. The scan takes about five minutes and is painless.

It works using waves of ultra sound to create a picture. Solid matter appears as white, whereas less solid matter, such as muscle and tissue, appear grey.

There is a fold of skin at the back of the baby's neck – the Nuchal Fold – and it is measured to assess the possibility that the baby may have Down's syndrome. A space measuring more than 2.5mm can be a high risk. If there is a possibility of Down's syndrome, your daughter will be offered further investigative tests.

This first scan will also reveal how many babies there are, that the heart is beating and that the measurements of the baby match your daughter's period of pregnancy.

Second trimester (weeks 13 to 28)

During this time your daughter's discomforts should ease and she should start to feel much better if she has been suffering. This will also be a time of greater energy and the pregnancy will begin to show.

Now would be a good time for her to get herself measured for a correctly fitted bra and, if the budget is not too tight, a small range of maternity wear to see her through the coming months.

During this period the baby's growth rate will accelerate and your daughter should expect to feel the first movements between 17 and 21 weeks. Some people report these movements as feeling like fish swirling about under the skin, others say it is like excess gas. Your daughter may have her own description for it.

By the end of this trimester, the baby will weigh about two pounds in weight and measure about 36cm.

Around week 20 or 21, your daughter will be invited for her next scan, which is a more thorough check-up.

The anomaly scan

This is a more detailed scan of the baby and the womb. The sonographer will check all the vital organs, including the baby's brain, measure its limbs, the amount of amniotic fluid and the position of the placenta. Your daughter may get to hear the baby's heart beating and she may even discover the sex of the baby at this stage if she wishes.

Common complaints

- ▒ Abdominal pain (from stretching ligaments).

- ▒ Backache.

- ▒ Bleeding gums.

- ▒ Constipation.

- ▒ Cravings.

- ▒ Insomnia.

- ▒ Nasal sensitivity.

- ▒ Pigmentation (the sun can make this more distinct).

- ▒ Piles.

- ▒ Stretchmarks.

- ▒ Sweating.

- ▒ Altered taste.

- ▒ Thrush.

'The sex of the baby can usually be determined at the second scan. Depending on how the baby is laying, it may not be possible to be a 100% sure. Some hospitals have a policy of not telling patients the sex of their baby.'

'Many alternative and complementary therapies can help relieve some of the discomfort associated with pregnancy. There are, however, special considerations and precautions to take when pregnant. It is essential, therefore, that anyone performing these therapies on your daughter is a qualified and registered practitioner.'

- Tiredness.

- Urinary infections.

- Vaginal discharge.

- Varicose veins.

- Visual disturbances.

You should ensure that your daughter is consuming a healthy diet and taking any prescribed tablets such as iron, especially if she is expecting more than one baby.

Anaemia

Anaemia is quite prevalent in pregnancy and even more so if the mother is very young. But what is anaemia?

Simply put, it is a reduction in the blood's ability to carry oxygen.

Your daughter's haemoglobin levels will be tested regularly and the medical team will hope for a result above 11g/dl.

If the results come back low, iron tablets may be prescribed. Symptoms of anaemia include fatigue, dizziness, fainting, headache and shortness of breath. Severe cases may experience chest pains.

During my last pregnancy, they found at my booking visit that my iron levels were low. In fact, only 7g/dl.

The midwife advised that I go immediately to hospital for a blood transfusion. I was admitted and given three pints of blood via an intravenous drip. My blood was tested again after the third pint had gone in; the results were better, though still low at 10g/dl. I was prescribed stronger iron tablets and then allowed home.

The third trimester (weeks 29 to 40)

In the final three months, your daughter should start preparing physically and mentally for the labour and birth. It is also important to assemble equipment and set up a nursery for the baby, if she is keeping it.

By weeks 36 to 40, the baby can weigh anything from five and a half pounds upwards, and measure about 20 to 22 inches. It can distinguish light and dark and can hear sounds.

Common complaints

- Braxton Hicks contractions (painless, practice contractions).
- Backache.
- Bleeding gums (maintain dental appointments).
- Constipation.
- Cramps.
- Cravings.
- Discomfort in bed.
- Fainting.
- Flatulence.
- Heartburn and indigestion.
- Incontinence.
- Insomnia.
- Increased dreams.
- Itching (anything severe needs to be checked).
- Frequency of passing urine.

- Nasal sensitivity.

- Oedema (swelling of the hands and feet).

- Pelvic discomfort.

- Pigmentation.

- Piles.

- Rashes.

- Rib pain.

- Shortness of breath.

- Stretchmarks.

- Sweating.

- Taste sensation.

- Thrush.

- Tiredness.

- Urine infection.

- Vaginal discharge.

- Varicose veins.

Your daughter may only experience one or two of the above, if any.

Other tests

As the pregnancy progresses, other tests may be required. The doctor or midwife will make your daughter fully aware of them and why they are being carried out. In as sensitive a manner as possible, you could discuss the implications with her of having a baby with some sort of disability.

AFP screening

AFP stands for alpha fetoprotein, a substance found in your daughter's blood during pregnancy. Testing the level of this will show whether your daughter's baby has a chance of having spina bifida or other neural tube defect. The levels fluctuate during the nine months but testing is usually done at around 17 weeks. The test results are not conclusive and simply indicate whether further investigations are required.

Amniocentesis

This is used to detect many conditions in the baby and involves passing a needle through your daughter's abdomen to collect a sample of amniotic fluid (water around the baby), which is then sent off for testing.

It may be offered if the chances of having a Down's syndrome baby seem high. It is performed in the 16th week of pregnancy, and can take up to two weeks for the results to come back as the cells have to be cultured.

The test can detect other abnormalities too, such as Tay Sach's disease and cystic fibrosis.

Occasionally, amniocentesis can cause infection, and there is a 1% risk of it leading to miscarriage.

CVS (Chorionic Villus Sampling)

This test is performed between 10 and 12 weeks, and takes a sample of cells that develop into the placenta (chorionic villi). The cells can be taken through the vagina or the abdomen. Results usually take a few days. Once again, the procedure carries about a 1% risk of miscarriage.

Waiting for the results

It can be hard waiting for these results. Emotions run high, especially if she's worried about how she might cope with a disabled baby or feels that the last thing she wants to do is have an abortion.

Most people assume when they are pregnant that everything will be fine, so it can be a shock to have to go through these procedures. Even when the results return and are normal, they may still worry about the possibility of the tests being wrong. They are only reassured when the baby is born.

It's easy to say, but try to relax and not worry too much. Worrying won't help you either way, so it's best to wait and see and then deal with the results when you know what they are.

Chapter Seven
The Birth

Hospital birth

Your daughter will inevitably be advised to have her baby in hospital and not try for a home birth, due to her young age. It is up to her how soon she wants to be admitted during the early stages of her labour, but it would probably be better if she went in as soon as the labour starts, as the medical team will want to monitor her and the baby closely.

Signs of early labour

- Intermittent short contractions.

- A show (when the mucus plug of the uterus comes away).

- Waters breaking.

- Sickness/diarrhoea.

- Dull backache.

If her waters break, make a note of the time and whether the water is clear or coloured. Then phone the midwife immediately. There is an increased chance of infection when the waters have gone and her temperature will need to be monitored.

Labour – the three stages

There are three distinct stages of labour. The first stage allows your daughter's cervix (neck of the womb) to dilate until it is fully open. The second stage involves pushing the baby out of the birth canal, and the third stage involves delivery of the placenta.

First stage

For the first stage, your daughter's cervix will have to thin out (efface) and dilate until it is fully taken up and open wide enough for the baby's head to pass through.

The rate of dilation of the cervix varies enormously, but on average, for a first time mother, this may be about 1cm per hour (10cms being the average size it has to dilate to).

She may be given drugs to strengthen her contractions and other drugs to provide pain relief.

Second stage

For the second stage, your daughter will have to push the baby out. Most hospitals allow about an hour for this (sometimes more for a first baby) if the mother and baby seem well and are coping with the delivery. If complications set in, they might suggest a ventouse or forceps delivery.

In the case of ventouse, a suction cup is placed on the baby's head and pulled on by the obstetrician. Forceps are metal instruments which are placed on the baby's head. The baby can then be pulled and lifted out.

If serious complications set in, she may be whisked into the operating theatre for an emergency caesarean section.

Third stage

For the third stage of labour, the expulsion of the placenta, your daughter can opt for a natural or managed stage.

'If your daughter asks you to be her birthing partner, there are many ways you can help and support her. Practical techniques like rubbing her back, encouraging her to breathe properly and providing cold/warm flannels will help her deal with the pain.'

Need2Know

If she opts for natural, the midwives will wait for the placenta to detach from the wall of the uterus on its own. If she wishes to have a managed stage, a drug will be injected into her thigh and the placenta delivered by gentle traction soon afterwards.

Decisions

It will be wise for your daughter to spend some time making a birth plan. This will help to plan her preferences for delivery. Let her decide:

- Her choice of birth partner.

- If she wants to move about during labour.

- What pain relief she might prefer, if any.

- What she would like to try and avoid (say an episiotomy).

- Whether she wants the baby handed to her straight away or not.

- Whether she wants a natural or managed third stage.

- Whether she wants to breast or bottle feed.

If she has been attending parentcraft classes, they will have gone over some of these points and she will have a good idea of what to expect during labour. Help her to find answers to as many of her questions as you can, because making the transition from teenager to mother can be a scary time.

Caesarean birth

There are many different reasons for having a caesarean section. It will be best if your daughter is made aware of these beforehand; why they happen and how. The operation is major abdominal surgery and should not be looked upon as an 'easy option' (despite what you read about 'too posh to push'!). Recovery can take weeks.

'Your daughter may choose to have the baby's father or a close friend as her birthing partner. Accepting that you cannot be present at this important time may not be easy for you. Try and remember that your daughter needs to do what is right for her.'

Why?

Some of the reasons for caesarean birth are as follows:

- Prolapse of the umbilical cord (baby's oxygen supply can be cut off).

- Low-lying placenta (risk of haemorrhage).

- Placenta praevia (the placenta is below the baby).

- Foetal distress (baby is short of oxygen).

- Pelvic disproportion (pelvis is too small).

- Infection.

- Failure of the cervix to dilate.

It may also be done in the following cases where the risks are calculated to be too great:

- The baby is breech.

- Multiple pregnancy.

How is it done?

The operation takes around 45 minutes, depending on the surgeon and how many babies there are. The baby is usually born within the first five minutes though, and the rest of the time is taken carefully stitching the various layers of the womb and abdomen.

Your daughter will be partly shaved and given anti-thrombosis socks to wear until she is up and about again.

Next, she will be taken to theatre (some surgeons or anaesthetists prefer the birth partner to wait outside initially) and given either an epidural or spinal block. Once this has been administered, her birth partner will probably be allowed into theatre to sit by her head. She will have a drip in her hand and a catheter to keep her bladder empty. She may also have an oxygen mask on her face. A screen will prevent her from seeing the actual surgery.

In certain cases, a general anaesthetic may be given. In this case, your daughter will be asleep, so her birth partner's presence is not so essential. However, some surgeons are quite happy for this person to be in theatre to experience the baby's birth.

The incision is usually horizontal within the bikini line, and dissolvable stitches are used.

I experienced a caesarean with my second pregnancy. The reason was that I was carrying twins and one of them was breech. The operation is quick and the medical staff may talk to you while they work, reassuring you about what is happening and when the baby or babies are about to be delivered. The majority of time is taken on the stitching afterwards.

Home birth

This is an option but will probably be advised against due to your daughter's age. If this is something she feels strongly about, it should be discussed with her medical team.

Post-natally

After the birth, your daughter will be encouraged to hold and feed her baby. It is wise to have chosen the method of feeding beforehand. If she wishes to breastfeed, the midwives will teach her how to latch the baby on successfully and how to break suction safely.

Your daughter may also be shown how to bathe, dress and change her baby's nappy before she leaves hospital.

Even when she is discharged, support from the midwives will be there in daily visits for up to 10 days (more if she feels she needs them). From then on, a health visitor will take over.

Emotions

Your daughter may have heard about the 'baby blues' or post-natal depression, but she might not be aware of having either of them. It could be up to those around her to make sure she is okay and to keep an eye out for her wellbeing. If signs of depression are spotted then her midwife, health visitor or GP should be informed.

Checklist

- Take any prescribed medicine.

- Eat healthily and wisely.

- Keep up all antenatal and scan appointments.

- Has she made a birth plan?

- Has she thought about feeding?

- Be aware of early labour signs.

- Be aware of what can happen during birth.

- Keep an eye out for the baby blues.

Chapter Eight

What Do Babies Need?

Requirements

There are certain items that are considered essential, and unfortunately baby equipment can be expensive. Below you will find lists of things the baby needs now, those required later, and luxuries that aren't necessary but are nice!

If budget is a problem, buy second hand or see if there are friends or family who are willing to lend your daughter some items. Certain items should not be second hand, however, such as a car seat, as they may be unsafe.

Essentials

- A place to sleep (a crib, cot or Moses basket).

- A car seat.

- Bedding.

- Nappies.

- Baby wipes/cotton wool.

- Nappy rash ointment.

- Buggy/pushchair.

- Feeding equipment (if not breastfeeding).

- Steriliser.

- Clothes (including hats/scratch mitts/socks, etc).

Stuff for later

- Bouncy chair.
- Highchair.
- Toys.
- Books.

Nice to have, but not necessary

- Muslin squares.
- Baby bath.
- Changing mat.
- Changing bag.
- Sling/backpack.
- Fitted sheets/cellular blankets.
- Separate soft towels for baby.
- Baby bath foam and soap.
- Blunt ended scissors.

What does your daughter need?

- Sanitary wear.
- Breast pads.
- Time to rest.
- Good food.
- Plenty to drink (especially if breastfeeding).
- A support network.

There are many magazines and books on the market that will tell you what you need for a new baby and mother, and yes it would be nice to have it all. We know the excitement of going round a store and thinking 'Ooh, look at that!' and buying extras. But it can be worth saving your money as a lot of new mothers find that some of their 'essential' extras don't get used at all.

Save your extra money to make sure your daughter's got a decent washing machine, because she'll be washing a lot of sheets and clothes.

Checklist

- Work out how much money you've got to buy the essentials.

- If people want to buy clothes, ask them for the next size up rather than newborn.

- Remember not to compromise on safety.

- Get a new car seat.

- Try not to impulse buy.

- Buy only what she needs.

'Many stores and baby goods companies offer mum-to-be clubs and schemes. These are a great way to get special offers, discounts and free samples.'

Chapter Nine
Life with a Baby

What is it like to be a mother?

Seeing the baby for the first time may be a bit of a shock for your daughter. She may have an image in her head of a chubby-cheeked baby, clean-skinned, plump and cute, with fluffy hair. In reality, a newborn baby is nothing like that.

Depending on the type of birth, the baby's head may be misshaped, especially if she had a ventouse delivery. The baby may look wrinkly and a bit purple or bruised. Their eyes may be puffy and swollen and the cord stump can look a little alarming!

Let her know that this will change over the next few days and soon enough she'll have the plump little baby she imagined.

Bonding

Bonding is spoken about quite compellingly by some, usually by the rich and famous who can't wait to tell the world how they fell in love instantly with their newborn. But this doesn't always happen. In fact, quite often, it doesn't.

If your daughter seems to be having difficulty, wondering why she isn't feeling all these emotions about her baby, try to reassure and support her. The time will come eventually, but this can take weeks or even months, especially if she suffers from post-natal depression.

Bonding will be easier if she holds and feeds the baby straight after delivery and is encouraged to carry out all the acts of care that a baby requires, such as dressing, bathing and nappy changing.

A baby can be demanding and it will be totally dependent on its mother. It will be understandable if your daughter feels a little overwhelmed by this responsibility at first, so help her, but also encourage her to do things for the baby herself.

Your daughter

Remember that whatever type of delivery your daughter had, she will be feeling exhausted and may be in some pain afterwards. Added to that, she may be feeling confused, upset, elated or delighted. You've got a very hormonal, exhausted teenager with a baby to care for.

Encourage her to accept any painkillers she may need and let her know that she shouldn't be afraid to ring her bell and ask for help. That is what the staff are there for, and they do it for all mothers, not just teenage ones.

Your daughter may be overwrought by emotions, so encourage her to express these and to talk. She may have concerns about the baby's father or her future. Talk to her. Get everything out into the open, then afterwards if she needs to sleep, let her do so.

Special Care Baby Unit (SCBU)

Sometimes after delivery, a baby may need to go to the special care unit. They may have a low-birth weight and/or be premature. There may be a few breathing problems, or the doctors may just feel that the baby needs observation for a few hours.

If this happens, reassure your daughter that this is not too unusual and that it would be best if she went to the SCBU to look around.

The equipment can seem frightening, but the staff will be happy to answer any questions she may have about what the machines and monitors are doing.

If your daughter wishes to breastfeed, she can probably still do so. Even if the baby is being fed by a tube into its stomach, she can express the milk.

Coming back home

Your daughter will probably feel exhausted and overwhelmed when she first brings her baby home. Her body will be undergoing enormous physical and hormonal changes that may leave her feeling confused and weepy. She may have moments of euphoria and wellbeing and then sink into exhaustion and be upset the next.

This is normal.

Help her as much as you can by encouraging her to sleep when the baby sleeps, to eat healthy foods and drink plenty of fluids, particularly if she is breastfeeding.

If she is very tired, try to limit the visitors over the first week by only letting those closest call in with their good wishes.

If the baby's father is involved, ask him to come as much as possible so that he can help with nappy changes and baby care, or he may even take the baby out for a walk in its pram.

Your daughter may or may not experience afterpains as the uterus shrinks back to its normal size. Breastfeeding can help with this and can also help to reduce bleeding from the womb (lochia).

She must use sanitary towels as tampons increase the risk of infection. Her midwife will have explained what to expect, but the flow should lessen as the days go by, slowly changing colour from red to pale brown. She should notify someone if she detects a smell or strange discharge, or if she passes any clots. If this happens or if the flow suddenly increases again, it can be a sign of infection.

Encourage her to empty her bladder frequently and not to be afraid of her first bowel movement. It can be painful, but won't split any stitches. Laxatives can be given by the midwife if really necessary.

'Try to limit the number of visitors in the early days. Your daughter needs time to rest and recover.'

'Too many visitors can also make it harder to start establishing a routine.'

Coping with stitches

If your daughter has stitches, they may well be uncomfortable for a few days until they dissolve. Her soreness will disappear and she can help by sitting in a warm bath every day and making sure she changes her sanitary wear frequently. During the first 10 days, a midwife will check her stitches to make sure these are healing well.

The baby

There is no one perfect way to care for a baby. With the first you are learning, often worrying about your choices and options. It can often be a case of trial and error. As your daughter gets to grips with being a mother, she may seem lacking in confidence as she finds her way through the exhausting first few days.

Make things as easy as possible by having all the equipment she needs close to hand. This includes nappy changing equipment and having drinks close by when she feeds her baby.

Make sure she knows how to test the water temperature before putting her baby into the bath. All of these things may seem obvious and simple, but when you're an overwhelmed young mother these little things can really help.

Being a mother

Being a parent is a huge, never-ending and sometimes thankless task. It involves giving a lot of yourself because the baby, or child, does most of the taking.

As time goes by, your daughter will hopefully become confident enough to take the baby out herself. If she feels that all she wants to do is stay inside, let her adjust to becoming a parent in her own time, but know your boundaries. You are the grandparent, not the parent. Help by all means, but don't take over unless she asks you to.

Try to help her establish a routine. Babies are soothed by learning and knowing what comes next. Sleeping, feeding and changing routines may help if your daughter is feeling exhausted by a fractious, highly vocal baby. If she changes her baby's nappy before every feed it will then be awake enough to feed properly. Find out what works in her situation and go with it, remembering that every baby and child is different.

Your daughter will receive support from her midwife for the first 10 days. She will then be signed off to a health visitor, who will check the baby's growth and discuss future plans such as immunisation and other support systems.

The health visitor will encourage your daughter to take her baby regularly to the clinic for a weigh-in and general checks. It is best to take advantage of these offers as it gives her the opportunity to seek professional help regarding any questions or worries that she may have. She is likely to meet other mothers and make friends at the clinic too.

Crying

Some babies cry all the time. It's a fact, and it often comes as a huge shock. It isn't necessarily because of something you're doing or not doing. There are certain things you can do, however, which may help:

- Check if the baby needs feeding/changing/winding.

- Take the baby out in its pram.

- Take the baby for a drive.

- Check with the doctor to see if the baby has colic.

- Check for cranial osteopathy (by a qualified practitioner).

A crying baby can grate on the nerves. If your daughter feels she just 'cannot take any more' then offer to look after the baby for an hour or two to give your daughter the break she needs.

'Find out if there is a local mother-and-baby group aimed specifically at younger mums. Your daughter will be able to get practical advice and support as well as meeting other young women in the same position as herself.'

Post-natal depression

Teenagers are prone to post-natal depression (PND), but this does not mean that your daughter will get it.

80% of women suffer from 'baby blues' and most get weepy around the third day after birth, when the milk comes in, but some women go on to develop post-natal depression.

PND can occur straight after the birth or even up to two years afterwards. If this happens to your daughter, she may not be aware of what is happening. She may believe she doesn't feel any different, but you'll be able to see the difference. Don't let her struggle on, trying to pretend that everything is alright. The earlier it's treated, the better. And ensure that there's no pressure on her to be the perfect mother, if such a thing exists!

Treatment may consist of tablets (anti-depressants) for a short time, or the opportunity to talk regularly to a counsellor or psychotherapist. Take your daughter to the GP if you suspect something more serious than 'baby blues' and get help for her. It will be better for her, the baby, you and all those around her.

PND signs

- Feeling low/crying.

- Loss of confidence/ability.

- Pessimistic/negative thoughts.

- No appetite/weight loss.

- Over-eating/weight gain.

- Feelings of panic.

- Mood swings.

- Exhaustion.

What to expect with a new baby

So what exactly will your daughter face in the next few uncertain weeks? She may have heard or read about what life is like with a baby. She may even imagine it to be a certain way, but she won't know for sure. So what are the facts?

Umbilical cord

The baby's umbilical cord can cause great concern to any parent, so it's best to know a little bit about it. Your daughter will be advised in hospital on how to care for the stump, and its appearance, but to summarise:

- In the first few hours, it is bluish-white and sealed with a peg-like clamp.

- It will dry out over the first few days and turn black.

- It will usually separate painlessly from the baby between seven to 10 days of the birth and fall away.

Some babies develop an umbilical hernia which looks like a small lump around the belly button. It can mostly be seen when the baby is crying or distressed. It is caused by weak abdominal muscles, allowing some of the internal bowel to push forward. Most of these hernias disappear within the first year and only a few ever need a surgical procedure.

My daughter had a large umbilical hernia that protruded through her navel to a length of five centimetres. It never bothered her and never caused any discomfort or pain. As she grew, the hernia shrank somewhat but never went away. She underwent a small operation at the age of four to close the hole in her abdominal muscles and remove some of the excess skin from her belly button. She came home after a few hours and has not had any problem since. If this happens, it is nothing to worry about, but being a mother, sometimes you cannot help but worry!

A baby's genitalia

When a baby is born, its genitals are often swollen and enlarged, and this can include the breast and nipple area. It is caused by a transfer of hormones from mother to baby in pregnancy. A baby girl may have a swollen vulva and can even pass a small 'period' within hours of the birth. Baby boys will often have a swollen scrotum. These occurrences will pass quite quickly and are nothing to worry about.

Birthmarks

There are many different types of birthmark. Some aren't noticeable at birth, developing years later, it seems.

The most common is called a stork-bite birthmark. It is located at the back of the neck, just at the edge of the hairline and will disappear within the first year of the baby's life. Stork-bite birthmarks have also been noticed on the face. They do not require treatment and will pass with time. Other birthmarks include:

- Port-wine stains.
- Strawberry marks.
- Mongolian blue spots.

Port-wine stains

These are caused by small blood vessels that have enlarged in the skin, causing bright red and/or purple marks on the skin. Port-wine stains can be found anywhere on the body or face and are permanent, removable only by laser treatment.

Strawberry marks

These are hardly noticeable at first. You see a tiny red dot and think nothing of it. They can quickly grow into a large lump, usually raised from the skin. Don't panic though. Strawberry marks tend to shrink and disappear by the child's second year of life.

Need2Know

Mongolian blue spots

These skin markings are usually of a blue/black colour and found at the base of baby's back or on its bottom cheeks. They tend to be seen more on dark-skinned babies, but fade naturally over time and require no treatment.

Bowel movements

To start with, babies may have odd-coloured, weird-looking bowel movements. If your daughter knows what to expect she shouldn't be alarmed.

Midwives will make sure that your daughter's baby has passed a motion before they leave hospital. This first bowel movement is usually a thick, tar-like, blackish/greenish, sticky substance. It is called meconium and is caused by what the baby swallowed while in the womb, along with any mucus. Bowel movements over the next few days will gradually change colour to green or brown. They may be quite frequent, often up to five dirty nappies a day.

Your daughter will soon notice that the bowel movement colour changes to a strange yellow colour and it is more liquid than solid. The texture and thickness of the bowel movement will depend upon whether the baby is being purely breastfed, bottle-fed or has mixed feeds.

Reflexes

The baby's reflexes will be checked while in hospital and by the midwife when she comes to visit. There are a number to check for:

- Moro reflex.

- Rooting reflex.

- Grasp reflex.

- Walking reflex.

- Stepping reflex.

Testing the moro reflex should only be performed by a midwife or doctor, as it involves 'dropping' the baby in a special gentle way.

Baby sounds

Apart from crying, there are many other sounds her baby will make. They are all quite normal and nothing to be worried about unless they seem excessive. They include snoring, sneezing, hiccupping and snuffling.

With snuffling, it may sound as if the baby has phlegm or mucus, and your daughter can get this checked out if she is worried. It usually occurs because a newborn baby's nose bridge is rather low and air being breathed in and out has to pass through small and narrow passages.

Jaundice

Many new born babies develop mild cases of jaundice which, with a little care and attention, clears up quite quickly. Jaundice can become serious if left untreated though.

This type of jaundice is not a disease so it is not catching. It is usually noticed when the baby is a day or so old.

What causes it?

Jaundice is caused by an excess of bilirubin, a pigment in the blood. The baby's skin develops a yellowish tinge and it cannot rid itself of the excess bilirubin quickly enough as the liver is not mature enough.

Treatment

Treatment for jaundice can be simple and quick if noted early and treated promptly. Usually this just consists of ensuring the baby is taking in adequate fluids, but short bursts of exposure to ultra-violet light or sunshine can help. If the jaundice becomes more serious then treatment in a special care baby unit is strongly advised. See your daughter's doctor for advice.

Picking up the baby

Make sure your daughter knows how to handle her baby correctly. No doubt the midwife will have gone into detail about how to support the baby's head but it helps to be reminded when she has to pick the baby up for the first time and she is on her own. Also, ensure she knows to support the length of the baby's body, holding it close to her own body. This will help the baby feel more secure.

Topping and tailing

A baby will not require a full bath every day, but will need 'topping and tailing'. Your daughter will need cooled boiled water, cotton wool and a soft towel to lay her baby on.

Starting at the top, she should gently wipe her baby's face, ensuring she uses separate pieces of cotton wool for each eye. This helps to avoid any infection passing from one eye to the other. She should gently wipe from the inner corner of the eye, out towards the ear. Then, with another piece of cotton wool, she should wipe clean the ears, both behind and on the outside. She should never poke anything inside her baby's ears.

Next comes cleaning the baby's hands and feet. With fresh cotton wool, gently clean the fingers, trying to clean the part between the fingers where dirt gathers easily and becomes sticky. This can be tricky, but don't force the fingers apart. Let her do what she can. Afterwards, dry the hands with a soft hand towel.

Repeat for the feet and toes.

Thirdly comes the nappy change. Wipe clean with cotton wool, making sure that all the creases have been checked. Apply anti-nappy rash cream and give the baby a clean nappy. If the baby is a boy, ensure that your daughter knows not to pull back the baby's foreskin. She may need to do this later but should discuss it with the midwife or doctor.

Cradle cap

Cradle cap is very common and is not a sign of something being wrong, or that your daughter hasn't cleaned the baby properly. If she washes the baby's scalp gently every day with baby shampoo and then uses a soft-bristled brush to gently brush away the cradle cap, it should soon disappear. Please advise her not to pick at the cradle cap, however tempting it may be. There are special cradle cap shampoos available from chemists and shops, but only use these if the cradle cap persists.

Giving baby a bath

This can be a little worrying if you've never bathed a baby. Your daughter may worry that she will drop the baby, or that the baby will cry. Like everything, she will improve with practise and her baby can learn to enjoy bath time.

Your daughter must first learn to test the water temperature. A baby cannot regulate its temperature like an adult and what may feel cool to us can be quite warm for a baby. The tried and tested method is for your daughter to stick her elbow in the water. She should be able to feel that the water is neither too hot nor too cold. Alternatively, she can use a proper bath thermometer. These are quite common and there are many different designs.

Next, she should remove the nappy as usual and wrap the baby in a large soft towel. Using cotton wool, she should clean the baby's face. Supporting the baby's body in one arm, she can use her other hand to shampoo and rinse the baby's hair.

Dry the baby's hair gently by softly rubbing with a towel, then unwrap the baby and gently lower into the bath. Support the baby's shoulder and neck with one hand (tucking fingers into the baby's armpit), and its bottom and legs with the other. Once the baby seems to feel confident, she can use one hand to gently dribble water over the chest, cleaning the baby's creases.

When the baby is clean and ready to come out, continue to support its shoulders and neck as before and, placing the other hand underneath the bottom and legs, lift from the water. Lay the baby on a towel and quickly wrap him up warmly.

'Your daughter may find it easier to use a specially-designed sponge or hammock which holds and supports the baby in the bath. This leaves both her hands free. They are not very expensive and you may even be able to pick up a second-hand one for a couple of pounds.'

Ensure the baby is dried thoroughly as any wetness can cause chafing and irritation. Put on a clean nappy and dress the baby. Talk reassuringly all the time so that the baby realises there is nothing to be worried about when bath time occurs.

Baby diarrhoea

Babies' bowel movements change frequently in colour and texture and sometimes your daughter may wonder whether all is normal. The changes could be due to something as simple as a different brand of formula, the heat or a new food.

If the stools are watery and have an increased offensive smell, and the baby seems a little 'off colour', then it would be wise for your daughter to consult her doctor. In healthy children and adults, diarrhoea is not usually dangerous. To a small baby, however, it has the potential danger to cause extreme dehydration very quickly. The doctor or midwife may check for dehydration by observing the baby's fontanelles, the two soft spots on the top and back of the baby's head. If the fontanelles are depressed, this can be a sign of dehydration and requires attention.

If your daughter notices a mild case of diarrhoea then she can carry on as normal. If she is breastfeeding, she can continue to do so. If she is using formula it can be wise to weaken this to half strength but using the same amount of water. Older babies can be given rehydration formulas, such as Dioralyte, but remember that diarrhoea can become serious, so it is best to err on the side of caution and seek medical advice.

If in doubt, ask questions.

If the diarrhoea is accompanied by vomiting in a young baby, the chance of dehydration is much higher, so always consult your doctor.

Nappy changing

A baby will need its nappy changed thousands of times and it's best to know how to do it correctly from the start. Nappies should be changed even if just wet because ammonia from stale urine can cause chafing and nappy rash.

Suggest to your daughter that she tries to stick to some routine, perhaps changing the nappy first thing in the morning, then after or before every feed, then again at bath time and once again before the baby is put down for the night. And have nappies to hand for those night changes!

Lay the baby flat on its back on a changing mat or old towel and remove the old nappy. Clean and wipe with cotton wool or wipes, always wiping from front to back. Holding the baby's ankles with one hand, gently lift the baby and slide the new, clean nappy underneath. Bring the front part up between the legs and fasten, checking for fit around the waist. If the umbilical stump is still present, make sure there is no chance that the nappy edge rubs against it and irritates. If the baby is a boy, remind your daughter that boys are notorious for weeing as soon as the nappy is removed!

Preventing nappy rash

Nappy rash can be kept to a minimum by following some basic rules. It can still appear occasionally, however, no matter how hard you try, especially if the baby has sensitive skin.

- Do not use soap on the baby's bottom as it removes natural skin oils.

- Remove nappies as soon as they become wet/dirty.

- Use a barrier cream.

- Leave the baby's bottom open to air as often as possible.

- Make sure the baby is dried properly after a bath.

- Use a barrier cream on noticeably red areas.

Choosing clothes

It can be very tempting to want to buy all the cute baby clothes when you go shopping. It's best to remind your daughter though that she needs to think of practicalities. Can what she has chosen be removed easily? Does it have

'If your daughter is considering cloth nappies, find out if your local council run a real nappy scheme. She may be able to get information, support and even a cash grant.'

easy nappy access? Will any of the fastenings chafe? Is any part of the item restrictive (toes and fingers need to be able to move)? Will it wash easily? Is it cotton or pure wool?

A baby will not care if it is wearing the latest designer clothes or the current fashionable colour. They just require comfort and warmth from clothes.

If your daughter gets the all-in-one stretch suits, remind her that when the baby gets bigger she can cut off the bootee part and get a few extra weeks of wear from the items, if money is tight.

Sleeping area

Babies sleep for a lot in the early weeks and it's best to have an established place for this. You need not spend lots of money decorating a nursery and buying the latest cot-bed combination. For the early days, your daughter can just put the baby in a Moses basket or use the carrycot part of her pram.

Never let the baby sleep for a long period of time in a car seat. This should never be used as a baby's bed.

The Moses basket can be quite portable if you're desperate for space, but eventually the baby will require a proper cot. Buy second hand if you wish, there are plenty of lovely ones on the market or on eBay, but *always* get a brand new foam mattress that has air holes.

The best cot to get is one with a drop side, making it easier to remove the baby for feeding and changing. A dropside also makes it easier for your daughter to roll over at night and give baby a reassuring touch if they are grizzling. Use cotton sheets and extra cellular blankets if it is particularly cold.

A thermometer can help to monitor the temperature of the bedroom. 18°C is best, and at this temperature she could use a sheet and two blankets, taking away layers if it gets warmer and vice versa.

A baby listener is great for a new, inexperienced mother. Your daughter will be able to keep in touch when she is in another room, and it will also save her from jumping up and running at the slightest grizzle. Baby listeners come in two parts, one part in the baby's room and the other, which can be attached to a belt or pocket, in the room where you are. There are many different varieties, either battery powered or mains, and some have indicator lights to show you the level of noise being generated by the baby, which can be very handy if your daughter has difficulty with her hearing.

Cot death

Cot death, also known as Sudden Infant Death Syndrome (SIDS), is when a baby suddenly dies for no apparent reason.

The cause of cot death is not known, although several risk factors have been identified. There is much advice on the subject and your daughter can ask her midwife or doctor if she has any particular questions or concerns. Basic suggestions are given below to help reduce the risks.

How can she reduce the risk?

- Ask your daughter not to smoke.

- Ask those around the baby not to smoke.

- Keep in smoke-free atmospheres as much as you can.

- Check the baby's temperature if it seems unwell.

- Do not use too many blankets.

- Do not tuck the blankets in.

- Allow the baby room for movement if it gets hot.

- Take an unwell baby to a doctor for a check-up.

- Put the baby to sleep on its back in the feet to foot position.

Feet to foot position

The feet to foot position means placing the baby at the bottom end of the cot so that its feet can just touch the footboard. This prevents the baby from snuggling down beneath the blankets, which could reduce airflow.

Smoking while pregnant appears to increase the risk of cot death. If your daughter smokes, encourage her to give up for the sake of her baby as well as herself (see section on smoking).

Chapter Ten

My Daughter's Education

Just because your daughter is about to have a baby, your discussions do not all have to be about pregnancy. Also of prime importance is the question of whether she wishes to continue her education.

If the answer initially is 'no', then be reassured that at least she can return to education at any time in the future, whether it's in one year or 10. But if she does want to continue her education after a period of 'maternity leave', then there are a couple of options open to her.

Statutory duty of the LEA (Local Education Authority)

LEAs have a duty to provide suitable education for any pupil of school age that becomes a parent, whether it is the mother or the father of a baby.

'Suitable education' must meet the individual need of the student regardless of their age, ability, aptitude and need. This includes pupils with special needs.

So what does this mean for your daughter?

It means that despite the pregnancy, the LEA and school *must* provide your daughter with an education tailored to her individual needs, no matter what. Even if your daughter has a Statement of Special Educational Needs, she should be treated in the same way as any other pupil at the school.

If your daughter is unable to attend school when she finds she is pregnant, the LEA is expected to provide her education, including setting and marking her work. The LEA will even provide free transport to her if they deem it necessary for her to attend school rather than learn at home.

What else?

The LEA may find your daughter a place at a Pupil Referral Unit (PRU) or other educational centre, or even choose to tutor her at home. Decisions about these options are made in consideration of individual circumstances.

A pregnant, school-age mother will remain on her school's register unless she has been excluded for another reason other than the pregnancy. (Your daughter cannot be expelled for getting pregnant.)

Be aware, however, that if your daughter has become pregnant while in Year 11, there may not be enough time for her re-integration after the birth. In this case the LEA's aim will be to encourage your daughter to pursue further education. (The Connexions service can provide more details in these situations.)

If you or your family are unable to help your daughter with childcare, she may be eligible for financial help so that she can continue her education. If both you and your partner work, you may be eligible to claim Working Families' Tax Credit for the care of your grandchild, and your daughter can claim Child Benefit.

Is my daughter 'in need'?

No. The fact that your daughter is pregnant below the age of 16, or is a young mother, does not necessarily make her a 'child in need'. If you feel that she needs extra help for whatever reason, she will need to be assessed by social services.

The school and your daughter

The school's aim will be to keep your daughter in education and the learning environment. If the head teacher believes the school is not a safe or suitable environment for her, this must be agreed by your daughter, you, the LEA and a Connexions advisor or Sure Start Plus advisor. (Sure Start Plus also supports the teenage father.)

Your daughter should inform the head teacher and the LEA about her pregnancy so that arrangements can be made for her continuing education. The head teacher, once informed, can then instruct other staff and pupils to handle the pregnancy sensitively and ensure that any bullies are dealt with in line with the school's bullying policy.

How much time off can she have?

Your daughter is entitled to no more than 18 weeks of authorised leave from school. This includes the period before birth and that afterwards.

If your daughter fails to return to school, she should still have access to support from them, the LEA and a Connexion's advisor who will help her return to education when she is ready.

Absences for antenatal classes or illness of the baby will be classified as authorised.

Friends

Your daughter's friends may react in a variety of ways, and it may be best to prepare your daughter for all eventualities.

Some friends may treat her as before, others may see her as someone to ridicule, while others may treat her with a sort of prestige. Let your daughter know that if bullying occurs it should be reported to her school and to you.

She will certainly learn who her real friends are. Unfortunately, if she finds this process upsetting, it is one of those times when there is no obvious answer. Give her the support she needs. Be there for her. You cannot control her friends.

My daughter is over 16

A popular option for continuing education can be distance learning, and there are many colleges and schools that offer home-learning at a price.

Choosing to study at home will depend on your financial circumstances. Your daughter may be entitled to a grant to pay for the course, or she could pay a small amount towards the tuition in instalments.

Though distance learning is a popular option, the loneliness of studying alone at home can itself cause problems:

- Finding a quiet place to study.

- Not being disturbed.

- No motivation without competition.

- Feelings of loneliness.

Taking exams

Your daughter can sit her GCSEs by registering with the examinations' board as an independent student. This can be done online, by telephone or post, but if she is educating herself through distance learning, these providers are likely to register her for exams at the appropriate times. (Individual institutions may vary.)

Future goals

It may be hard to make decisions while caring for a new baby, but it is worth your daughter thinking about her future and any career she may have in mind.

Will having the responsibility of a child interfere with her plans? Or, if she has chosen abortion or adoption, will these choices affect her future goals?

Spend time with your daughter to talk about the possible options, but do not rush this process. This is her future. She should be thinking about it seriously and not assuming that everything will work out alright. While it may well do, it's more likely to do so if carefully planned.

Childcare

If your daughter chooses to go back to school, then the question of who cares for the baby will arise. Will she expect you to look after the baby? What about your own job? Are you happy to put your life on 'hold' until she finishes her education? If yes, then it isn't a problem. But what if the answer is no?

Is there someone else she trusts who could look after the baby?

If she has chosen distance education and is learning at home, does she feel that she will be able to achieve what she wishes while being fully occupied with the baby too? What if the baby has colic and cries a lot? Will she be able to cope with tiredness and constant interruptions?

Checklist

- Decide whether to continue her education now or later.

- Choose which option of schooling is best.

- If distance learning, make sure she's registered with the exam provider.

- Think of how her choices may affect her future.

- Arrange suitable childcare.

- Discuss what she wants for the future.

'Care to Learn is a scheme which allows teenage parents to claim childcare and travel costs if they are at school or college. Find out more at www.dfes.gov.uk/caretolearn or by calling 0845 6002809.'

Chapter Eleven

Legal Matters

What is the law?

Certain laws govern everybody, but there are specific ones which relate to parents and children, so let's start at the beginning.

Registering a birth

At the time of writing, a parent is allowed up to six weeks to register a child being born. This must be done with the District Registrar for Births, Marriages and Deaths.

A birth has to be registered in the district where the baby was born, and register offices are usually conveniently situated next to the hospital or in a city centre, so are easy to find.

The registrar will ask simple questions such as the date, time and place of birth and the child's name, as well as its parents' names and addresses. The baby's father cannot register the birth on his own, your daughter has to be present. His details will only be included if:

■ He wishes it and your daughter agrees.

■ Your daughter asks for his details to be added and he has made a statutory declaration that he is the father.

■ There is a court order showing that he is the father.

A child does not necessarily take its father's surname. Children can be registered with your daughter's surname or hyphenated with the father's.

Can you alter the register later?

Yes. If the mother consents to an alteration, or a court order proves that the named male is the father of the baby, the details can be changed or added. The register can also be changed within the first year if the parents decide to change the name of the baby or they discover that other details are wrong.

Adopted children

By the time a child is adopted it already has a birth certificate which has been registered by the natural mother of the child. When an adoption procedure goes through, a new certificate is drawn up which gives the date of birth, the possible new name and the names and address of the adoptive parents. This new certificate will become the official birth certificate and the old one will be null and void.

There are two types of birth certificate:

- The short one which gives details of the child but no mention of the parents.

- The longer certificate which contains all parental details.

Both types are legally valid.

When an adopted child reaches the age of 18, they are allowed to trace their natural parents' names through the official register: General Register Office, PO Box 2, Southport, Merseyside, PR8 2JD. Tel: 0151 471 4816.

The adoptive children's register was created by the Children's Act in 1989. This gives blood relatives the opportunity to put their names on the register as a point of contact when the adoptive child wishes to get in touch with his/her birth family. However, this register can only be used by the adopted child. If your daughter has given her baby for adoption, she cannot use this register to find out her child's whereabouts or new name. It is totally confidential and for the adoptee only.

If the baby has already been taken into care then the Local Authority (LA) can place the child up for adoption. Your daughter, in this situation, can refuse to have her child adopted, but the authority can apply to the court to make a 'freeing order'.

Who can adopt the child?

- A married couple (both 21 or over).

- A parent and step-parent.

- A single person (over 21 years).

The British Association for Adoption and Fostering (BAAF) issues a monthly newsletter for families interested in adopting. It is called *Be My Parent*, and you can request a copy by telephoning 020 7593 2060/2061/2062.

Unmarried parents

At the time of writing, 40% of children in the UK were born out of wedlock. These days, illegitimacy no longer caries the stigma it used to.

The Family Law Reform Act 1987 gives children the right to claim maintenance from their father.

If your daughter decides not to marry the baby's father then she has sole parental responsibility for her child, along with all the legal rights and duties inherent in that. But if the father wishes to be involved and have some say in the upbringing and future of his child, he must acquire parental responsibility. To get this, he must:

- Gain your daughter's agreement.

- Apply to the court.

- Be appointed guardian of the child if your daughter has died.

Parental responsibility

If your daughter agrees to share parental responsibility with the baby's father, they must both sign a form from the court to make this effective in the eyes of the law. Their signatures must be witnessed by a court official and they will have to provide proof of their identity.

Either your daughter or the baby's father can then register this form with the:

Principal Register of the Family Division
First Avenue House, 42-49 High Holborn, London, WC1V 6NP.

This will not cost anything.

Your daughter would be advised to think carefully about taking such a huge step because she will be giving the baby's father an opportunity to have a say in the child's life up to and including the age of 18. Does she feel that she will be able to maintain a friendly line of communication with him so they can meet regularly to agree decisions on their child's future? Can she foresee them being able to communicate amicably?

If your daughter refuses to let her baby's father have parental responsibility, he is allowed to apply for it on his own. If he has to take this route, consider whether it would set foundations for a peaceful relationship between the two? He will have to prove to the court that he is a good father, that he is committed and that they have a solid relationship.

The court will only agree to approve his parental right if they think it is in the best interest of the child. A parental responsibility order does not legally make him the father of the child, it will only give him a legal connection.

Paternity

Perhaps there is question over who is the father of the baby. Perhaps the issue over who the father is has never been resolved and there is more than one party claiming to be 'the one'.

Where paternity is disputed, responsibility for the father and maintenance for the child cannot be claimed unless paternity has been proven, and a DNA test is required for this.

Samples will be taken from the mother, the baby and the possible fathers. A court cannot order a man to take a paternity test, but if he refuses then the court can assume that he is the father.

If your daughter refuses to let samples be taken from the child, there is nothing anyone can do about it.

Finances

For information about which benefits your daughter and her child is entitled to it is best to contact someone who can inform you about this on an individual basis: The National Council for One Parent Families. Tel: 0800 018 5026 (Free helpline).

Maintenance

The father of a baby is required to provide for his child whether he is married to the mother or not, and no matter what the state of their relationship was when the child was conceived. The Child Support Agency can assess how much he needs to pay within his own limitations and they have the power to enforce payment.

If the baby's father is raising the child and has sole parental responsibility, he can make a claim for child support from your daughter.

Abortion

The father of the baby cannot prevent your daughter from having an abortion. Nor can you, the teenager's parent, prevent an abortion.

Guardians

Your daughter can appoint a guardian for her child in the case of her death via a will or statement in writing. The guardian would then have full parental responsibility as if they were the biological parent.

Only the mother can appoint a guardian if she is not married, unless the father has been given parental responsibility. If he does not have this, he would have no rights or responsibilities in the child's life if your daughter were to die.

Education

The Education Act ensures that parents make certain their children are educated and that LEAs provide suitable schools in populated areas.

A child is of school age from the school year they turn five until the school year they turn 16. During those years, a child must receive a suitable education either at school or at home.

Education is compulsory, not school

If you choose to educate a child at home, be aware that the Local Authority (LA) can challenge the quality of that education. Parents then have two weeks to prove that the education is suitable. Parents who wish to teach their own children do not have to be qualified teachers, but it helps if they are, especially if the Local Authority (LA) decides to challenge their suitability.

Chapter Twelve

Contraception

Once the pregnancy and birth are over you may worry that it could all happen again. It certainly wouldn't be a good idea for your daughter to get pregnant again immediately, so it may be a good idea to discuss birth control with her, even if she insists that she won't get pregnant.

What choices are open to her?

There are many choices of birth control open to everyone, and these options are listed below:

- Abstinence.
- Condoms.
- The (combined) pill.
- Natural methods.
- Caps/diaphragms.
- Injections.
- Implant.
- Contraceptive skin patch.
- IUDs & IUS.
- Emergency contraception.

So let's look at each of these in turn and discuss the pros and cons.

'It has been estimated that as many as 20% of births to mothers under 18 are second or subsequent pregnancies.'

Abstinence

Abstinence is the only fully effective way of avoiding pregnancy and sexually transmitted infections.

Do you know if your daughter will be celibate? Do you feel you can trust what she has said? If so, that's great, but abstinence requires a great deal of control, especially if you have a partner with whom you've already been sexually active. Therefore, it would be advisable to think of another method if you, or she, feels that she wouldn't be able to say 'no'.

Condoms

Condoms are the only method of contraception which also provide protection against STIs. Used correctly, they are very reliable.

Condoms are available free of charge from all sorts of places, including many youth centres and young people's services. They are also available from family planning and sexual health clinics; again free of charge. Almost all chemists and supermarkets sell condoms and many public facilities have condom vending machines.

There is no denying that condoms do require willpower and commitment. They must be used every time, at the right time, and must be on correctly. It can also be difficult, especially for young people, to discuss – and if necessary insist on – using condoms with their partner. There is, however, a good deal of information and support available for young people on this subject. You could also take the opportunity of reading leaflets, checking websites, etc with your daughter.

Although less well-known than the male condom, a female condom is also available. These are often referred to by the brand name 'Femidom' and can be obtained from most places that give out male condoms (few retail outlets stock the female condom).

The female condom is made of latex and is placed inside the vagina. It acts as a barrier, preventing sperm and STIs getting through. Again, effectiveness is dependant upon proper use but, used correctly, the female condom offers protection from both pregnancy and STIs.

The clear advantage of the female condom is that it can be put in place before a sexual activity has started. There is no need to interrupt 'proceedings' and your daughter does not have to rely on the co-operation of her partner as much as with male condoms.

Further information on condom use and safer sex is available from www. condomessentialwear.co.uk.

The (combined) pill

The pill is a very effective method of contraception. In order to get maximum protection, however, it must be taken consistently.

While the pill does not provide any protection against STIs, it can be used in conjunction with condoms. This can be a very effective way of protecting against both pregnancy and STIs.

There are other varieties of contraceptive pill such as Marvelon, Cilest and many others. These are taken once a day, at the same time, for three weeks. After those three weeks your daughter goes seven days pill-free. During this time she has a 'period', which is actually a withdrawal bleed from the drop in hormone level, before starting the next three weeks of pills.

There are many myths surrounding the use of oral contraceptives, such as the possibility of weight gain, nausea, etc. In reality, side effects are very rare and can usually be eliminated by switching the particular brand taken.

In some circumstances, when breastfeeding for example, women are prescribed with the POP pill which contains progestogen only.

The POP pill works slightly differently to the combined pill and is taken every day. There is no seven day break and periods may not be as regular as with the combined pill.

Legally, a 14-year-old can have the contraceptive pill prescribed by a doctor without her parent's consent, so if your daughter decides to take the pill this would not pose a legal problem. For more information about the pill, read *The Pill – An Essential Guide*.

Natural methods

Essentially, natural family planning involves observing and recording the body's natural indicators of fertility. These include body temperature, cervical mucus and menstrual cycle length. Sex is then avoided (or condoms used) when she is most likely to be fertile.

Natural family planning can be very effective but it needs to be used properly and should ideally be taught by a specialist natural family planning teacher.

If sex is avoided totally during fertile periods, rather than using condoms at this time, the natural family planning is acceptable to all religious faiths.

Caps/diaphragms

There are a number of types of caps and diaphragms. They work by sitting inside the vagina and covering the entrance to the womb. This helps stop sperm getting through. To be most effective, they should be used with a spermicide.

A woman needs to have the correct size and shape cap/diaphragm, so an initial fitting must be carried out by a doctor or nurse. Once she has the right fitting, a woman puts the cap in place each time she has sex. Like the female condom, a cap/diaphragm can be put in place before sexual activity starts.

Injections

The most common contraceptive injection is Depo-Provera. It is administered by a small injection, usually in the bottom, once every three months.

The distinct advantage of contraceptive injections is that effectiveness does not rely on remembering to take a pill every day. One injection, every three months, will provide on-going protection. Again, injections can be combined with condoms for protection against STIs.

Some women have reported side effects such as weight gain or irregular periods when using Depo-Provera but, for many, the possible disadvantages are out-weighed by the convenience and effectiveness of this method.

Implant

Becoming increasingly popular is the contraceptive implant, 'Implanon'. About the size of a matchstick, this is placed under the skin on the arm, using local anaesthetic. It is completely invisible and releases the hormone progestogen which prevents conception for three years.

Contraceptive patches

The contraceptive patch available in the UK is called Evra. It is a small, beige patch that is placed on the skin.

Evra releases progestogen and estrogen into the body, working much the same way as the combined pill. Unlike the pill, however, the hormones are released directly into the bloodstream so it is not affected by diarrhoea or vomiting. Patches are only changed once a week so it may be easier to remember than the pill.

Some women may experience temporary side effects with patches (nausea, headaches, breast tenderness), but these should stop within a few months.

IUDs & IUS

An IUD is a copper and plastic, t-shaped device which is inserted in the womb. Essentially, it works by causing an increase in white blood cells in the cervix, which prevents sperm getting through.

An IUD gives immediate protection against pregnancy and lasts for several years. Two soft strings hang from the device into the top of the vagina, allowing the user to check it is still in place at any time.

Some women may experience heavy or prolonged periods with an IUD, but there are many advantages of this 'fit it and forget it' method of contraception. It should be remembered, however, that IUDs do not protect against STIs.

The IUS is similar to an IUD in that it is t-shaped and placed inside the womb. There is only one type available, called the Mirena.

The Mirena releases a steady stream of the hormone progestogen and can be left in place for five years.

Both IUDs and the IUS can be easily removed if a pregnancy is desired.

Emergency contraception

Emergency contraception is available in two forms: a hormonal pill and IUDs.

The emergency contraceptive pill is often known as 'the morning after pill.' In reality, however, it can be taken up to 72 hours after sex, although it is most effective when taken as soon as possible.

It works by giving a high dose of hormones, similar to the pill, in single tablet form. For this reason it is not suitable as a regular method of contraception. A small number of women may experience nausea when taking the emergency contraceptive pill.

There are many places where the E.C.P. is available free of charge including doctors, walk in centres and sexual health clinics. It can also be bought over-the-counter in pharmacies.

The morning after pill used to be two pills that were taken 12 hours apart, but nowadays it is just the one pill. There are side effects, which include sickness and/or nausea, but these will not apply to everybody who takes it.

This contraception is available at the chemist. You no longer have to go to your doctor for the prescription.

IUD

The section above gives details of IUDs as long-term contraception. They can also be used, however, as emergency contraception.

An IUD can be fitted up to five days after unprotected sex and can then be left in place for on-going contraception.

Overview

As an overview on contraception, you can use any of the above regularly (except the morning after pill), but if you want to make sure your daughter avoids the possibility of infection then she should also use condoms.

Condoms can be used as well as one of the others to protect from pregnancy and infection. Of course, the only perfect way is to avoid having sex altogether. Not always a popular choice!

You cannot watch your daughter 24 hours a day and nobody would expect you to. You could maybe help her to gain a level of maturity and responsibility; after all, she has had a baby, whether she has kept it or not. So along with the professionals, give her as much information and options as you can so that she can choose for herself. There are consequences to every choice and we each have to live with those.

Checklist

- Discuss future contraceptive choice.

- Decide which method would be best.

- Talk things over at a family planning clinic or with her doctor.

- Make sure she understands her choices.

- Find out more by visiting local services or using young people's websites.

In conclusion

Hopefully this book has given you a baseline of knowledge to help you face the challenges of your daughter's pregnancy.

You may be having a grandchild as a result, or you may not.

Either way, your young, teenage daughter is/was pregnant and the issues are on-going whatever decisions are being made.

Keep the lines of communication open. Make sure she knows that you are 'there for her' and that she will have your support and guidance no matter what she has to face.

After all, that's what parents do.

They love their children.

They protect them.

And that is exactly what you have tried to do.

Help List

Action on Smoking and Health
102 Clifton Street, London, EC2A 4HW
Tel: 020 7739 5902
www.ash.org.uk
enquiries@ash.org.uk

The British Association for Adoption and Fostering
Saffron House, 6-10 Kirby Street, London, EC1N 8TS
Tel: 020 7421 2600
www.baaf.org.uk
Mail@baaf.org.uk

British Epilepsy Association
New Anstey House, Gate Way Drive, Yeadon, Leeds, LS19 7XY
Tel: 0113 210 8800 (UK)
www.epilepsy.org.uk
Helpline@epilepsy.org.uk
Helpline 0808 800 5050

British Pregnancy Advisory Service (BPAS)
4th Floor, Amec House, Timothy's Bridge Road, Stratford-Upon-Avon, CV37 9BF
www.bpas.org/
Tel: 0870 365 5050

Diabetes UK
Central Office, Macleod House, 10 Parkway, London, NW1 7AA
Tel: 020 7424 1001
www.diabetes.org.uk

Info@diabetes.org.uk

FPA
50 Featherstone Street, London, EC1Y 8QU
Tel: 0845 122 8690
www.fpa.org.uk

Miscarriage Association
c/o Clayton Hospital, Northgate, Wakefield, West Yorkshire, WF1 3JS
Tel: 01924 200799 (Mon-Fri, 9am-4pm)
www.miscarriageassociation.org.uk

QUIT
Ground Floor, 211 Old Street, London, EC1V 9NR
Quitline: 0800 00 22 00
NHS pregnancy smoking helpline: 0800 169 9169
www.quit.org.uk
Tel: 020 7251 1551

NCT (National Childbirth Trust)
Alexandra House, Oldham Terrace, Acton, London, W3 6NH

Tel: 0870 770 3236
www.nct.org.uk

NHS Direct
Tel: 0845 4647
www.nhsdirect.nhs.uk

Association for Post-Natal Illness
145 Dawes Road, Fulham, London, SW6 7EB

Tel: 020 7386 0868
www.apni.org

Association of Breastfeeding Mothers
PO Box 207, Bridgwater, Somerset, TA6 7YT
Helpline: 0870 401 7711
www.abm.me.uk
Info@abm.me.uk
Counselling@abm.me.uk

CRY-SIS
BM Cry-Sis, London, WC1N 3XX
Helpline: 0845 122 8669
www.cry-sis.org.uk/
Info@cry-sis.org.uk

La Leche League
Tel: 020 7242 1278 (24 hours)

MAMA (Meet-A-Mum-Association)
54 Lillington Road, Radstock, BA3 3NR
Helpline: 0845 120 3746 (7pm-10pm, weekdays)
www.mama.co.uk

Gingerbread
307 Borough High Street, London, SE1 1JH
Tel: 020 7403 9500
www.gingerbread.org.uk
advice@gingerbread.org.uk

BLISS (Baby Life Support Systems)
2nd & 3rd Floors, 9 Holyrood Street, London Bridge, London, SE1 2EL
Tel: 020 7378 1122

www.bliss.org.uk
Information@bliss.org.uk

Foundation for the Study of Infant Deaths
Artillery House, 11-19 Artillery Row, London, SW1P 1RT
Tel: 020 7233 2090
www.sids.org.uk

Multiple Births Foundation
Hammersmith House (Level 4), Queen Charlotte & Chelsea Hospital,
Du Cane Road, London, W12 0HS
Tel: 0208 383 3519
www.multiplebirths.org.uk
info@multiplebirths.org.uk

TAMBA (Twins and Multiple Births Association)
2 The Willows, Gardner Road, Guildford, GU1 4PG
Tel: 0870 770 3305
Twinline: 0800 138 0509

Websites for teenagers & parents

www.brook.org.uk

www.ruthinking.co.uk

www.fpa.org.uk

www.mariestopes.org.uk

www.bpas.org

www.parentlineplus.org.uk

www.teenagepregnancyunit.gov.uk

www.dfes.gov.uk/schoolageparents

www.dfes.gov.uk/caretolearn

www.connexions-direct.com

Telephone numbers and helplines

Sexwise

Tel: 0800 28 29 30 (free, confidential advice)

Working Families Tax Credits

Tel: 0845 609 5000

Adoption Information Line

Tel: 0800 783 4086 (9am-9pm, except bank holidays)

Talk Adoption

Tel: 0808 808 1234 (Tues-Fri, 3pm-9pm)

Marie Stopes Aftercare Line

Tel: 0845 122 1441 (24 hours)

Available Titles

Drugs A Parent's Guide
ISBN 978-1-86144-043-3 £8.99

Dyslexia and Other Learning Difficulties
A Parent's Guide   ISBN 978-1-86144-042-6 £8.99

Bullying A Parent's Guide
ISBN 978-1-86144-044-0 £8.99

Working Mothers The Essential Guide
ISBN 978-1-86144-048-8 £8.99

Teenage Pregnancy The Essential Guide
ISBN 978-1-86144-046-4 £8.99

How to Pass Exams A Parent's Guide
ISBN 978-1-86144-047-1 £8.99

Child Obesity A Parent's Guide
ISBN 978-1-86144-049-5 £8.99

Sexually Transmitted Infections
The Essential Guide   ISBN 978-1-86144-051-8 £8.99

Alcoholism The Family Guide
ISBN 978-1-86144-050-1 £8.99

Divorce and Separation The Essential Guide
ISBN 978-1-86144-053-2 £8.99

Applying to University The Essential Guide
ISBN 978-1-86144-052-5 £8.99

ADHD The Essential Guide
ISBN 978-1-86144-060-0 £8.99

Student Cookbook - Healthy Eating The Essential Guide
ISBN 978-1-86144-061-7 £8.99

Stress The Essential Guide
ISBN 978-1-86144-054-9 £8.99

Single Parents The Essential Guide
ISBN 978-1-86144-055-6 £8.99

Adoption and Fostering A Parent's Guide
ISBN 978-1-86144-056-3 £8.99

Special Educational Needs A Parent's Guide
ISBN 978-1-86144-057-0 £8.99

The Pill An Essential Guide
ISBN 978-1-86144-058-7 £8.99

Diabetes The Essential Guide
ISBN 978-1-86144-059-4 £8.99

To order our titles, please give us a call on **01733 898103**,
email **sales@n2kbooks.com**, or visit **www.need2knowbooks.co.uk**

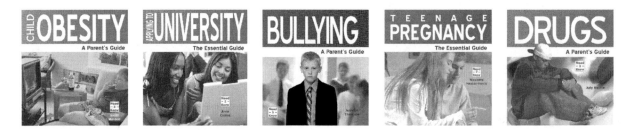

Need - 2 - Know, Remus House, Coltsfoot Drive, Peterborough, PE2 9JX